Build Muscle.
Stay Lean.
Get Stronger.

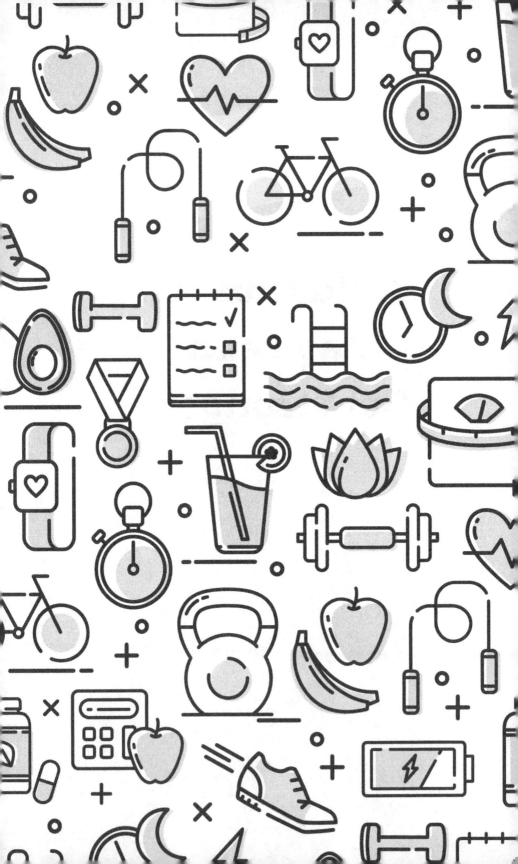

Build Muscle.
Stay Lean.
Get Stronger.

A Daily Food and Exercise Journal
to Track your Fitness Goals

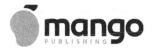

Mango Publishing

CORAL GABLES

For permission requests, please contact the publisher at:

Mango Publishing Group
2850 Douglas Road, 2nd Floor
Coral Gables, FL 33134 USA
info@mango.bz

For special orders, quantity sales, course adoptions and corporate sales, please email the publisher at sales@mango.bz.
For trade and wholesale sales, please contact Ingram Publisher Services at customer.service@ingramcontent.com or +1.800.509.4887.

Medical citations:

"Building Muscle Simplified: Not as Complicated as You Think," ISSA Online, last accessed 10/9/2019, www.issaonline.com/blog/index.cfm/2018/building-muscle-simplified-not-as-complicated-as-you-think

Dr. Erin Nitschke, "How Muscle Grows," Ace Fitness, last updated 8/30/2017, www.acefitness.org/education-and-resources/lifestyle/blog/6538/how-muscle-grows?topicScope=exercise-science

Build Muscle. Stay Lean. Get Stronger: A Daily Food and Exercise Journal to Track your Fitness Goals

Library of Congress Cataloging
ISBN: (p) 978-1-64250-157-5 | (e) 978-1-64250-156-8
BISAC: HEA007000, HEALTH & FITNESS / Exercise / General

Printed in the United States of America

Fitness

noun

fit·ness (fit-nəs)

Definition of *fitness*

1: the quality or state of being fit

Merriam-Webster

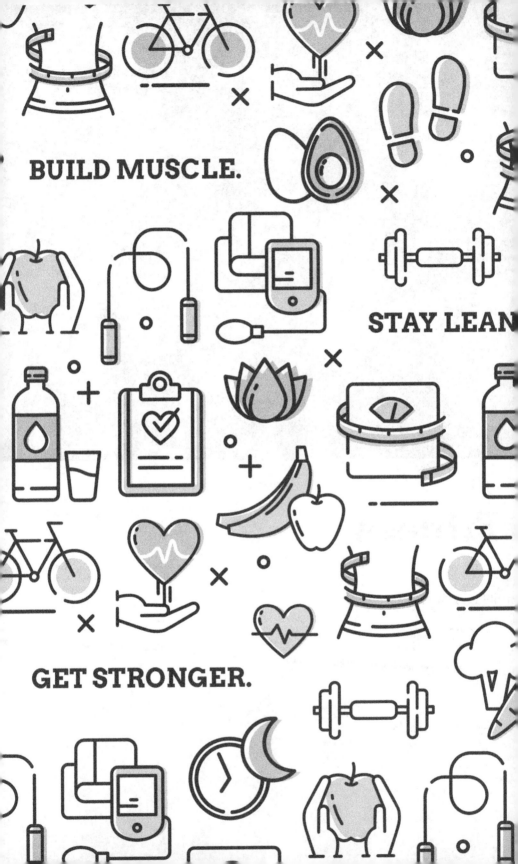

Before We Get Started...

It is important to understand how muscle is built and what that means in relation to a healthy body. While it may seem obvious, between keto diets, paleo fads, and fasting regimens, this type of information can get misconstrued. When it comes to your body's overall health, the keys are to have a strong heart, healthy organs and blood flow, and energy to sustain your weight.

But what does that mean exactly? Fat can provide fuel, and some people can eat fries by the carton and not gain a pound.

Because all our bodies are unique and react to foods and exercise routines differently, it is impossible to have a one-size-fits-all plan. What we do know is that it is important for everyone to partake in regular resistance training and cardiovascular training for better health. But before starting any new exercise regimen, you should consult your physician.

Fitness Goals

Fitness Goals

List any goals you want to **achieve every day** as you embark on this new journey.

EAT CLEANER AND HEALTHIER

EXERCISE

SLEEP (   ) HOURS

DRINK (   ) CUPS OF WATER

_____

_____

_____

_____

_____

Fill in the heart around **each day** that you achieve your goals.

	Sunday	Monday	Tuesday	Wednesday	Thursday	Friday	Saturday
Week 1	♡	♡	♡	♡	♡	♡	♡
Week 2	♡	♡	♡	♡	♡	♡	♡
Week 3	♡	♡	♡	♡	♡	♡	♡
Week 4	♡	♡	♡	♡	♡	♡	♡
Week 5	♡	♡	♡	♡	♡	♡	♡
Week 6	♡	♡	♡	♡	♡	♡	♡
Week 7	♡	♡	♡	♡	♡	♡	♡
Week 8	♡	♡	♡	♡	♡	♡	♡
Week 9	♡	♡	♡	♡	♡	♡	♡
Week 10	♡	♡	♡	♡	♡	♡	♡
Week 11	♡	♡	♡	♡	♡	♡	♡
Week 12	♡	♡	♡	♡	♡	♡	♡
Week 13	♡	♡	♡	♡	♡	♡	♡

Let's Get Moving!

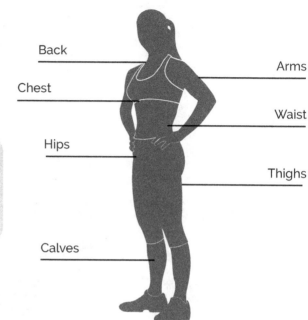

Back

Arms

Chest

Waist

Hips

Thighs

Calves

Weight: _____

Heart Rate: _____

Blood Pressure: _____

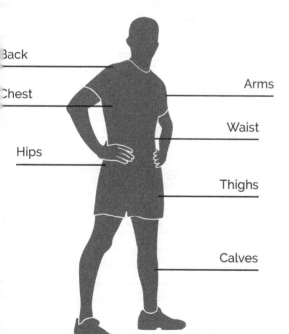

Back

Arms

Chest

Waist

Hips

Thighs

Calves

Weight: _____

Heart Rate: _____

Blood Pressure: _____

DAY (1)   How many hours of sleep did I get?

Breakfast	Lunch	Dinner

Snacks

8oz 16oz 24oz 32oz 40oz 48oz 56oz 64oz

Macros

Carbs:

Protein:

Energy Levels

Fats:

Total Calories:

Resistance Workout Tracker

Exercise	Reps	Set	Weight	Notes

Cardio Workout Tracker

Exercise	Reps	Set	Weight	Notes

Notes

How many hours of sleep did I get?

Breakfast

Lunch

Dinner

Snacks

8oz 16oz 24oz 32oz 40oz 48oz 56oz 64oz

Macros

Carbs:

Protein:

Fats:

Total Calories:

Energy Levels

Resistance Workout Tracker

Exercise	Reps	Set	Weight	Notes

Cardio Workout Tracker

Exercise	Reps	Set	Weight	Notes

Notes

DAY 3   How many hours of sleep did I get?

Breakfast	Lunch	Dinner

Snacks

8oz 16oz 24oz 32oz 40oz 48oz 56oz 64oz

Macros

Carbs:

Protein:

Energy Levels

Fats:

Total Calories:

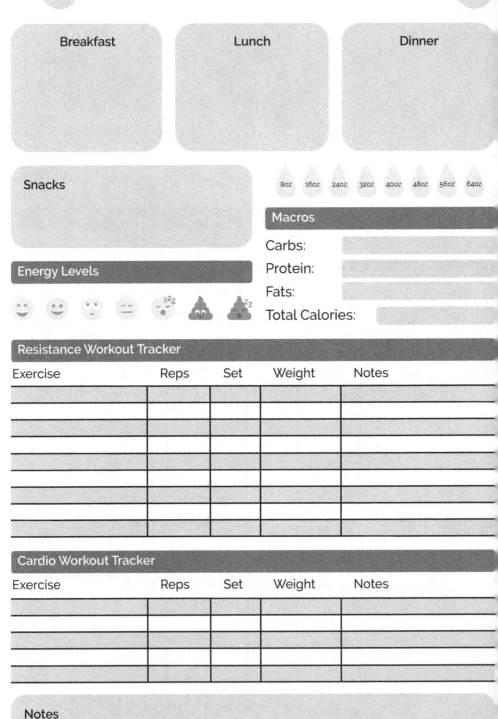

Resistance Workout Tracker

Exercise	Reps	Set	Weight	Notes

Cardio Workout Tracker

Exercise	Reps	Set	Weight	Notes

Notes

How many hours of sleep did I get?

Breakfast

Lunch

Dinner

Snacks

8oz 16oz 24oz 32oz 40oz 48oz 56oz 64oz

Macros

Carbs:

Energy Levels

Protein:

Fats:

Total Calories:

Resistance Workout Tracker

Exercise	Reps	Set	Weight	Notes

Cardio Workout Tracker

Exercise	Reps	Set	Weight	Notes

Notes

DAY 5

How many hours of sleep did I get?

Breakfast

Lunch

Dinner

Snacks

8oz 16oz 24oz 32oz 40oz 48oz 56oz 64oz

Macros

Carbs:

Energy Levels

Protein:

Fats:

Total Calories:

Resistance Workout Tracker

Exercise	Reps	Set	Weight	Notes

Cardio Workout Tracker

Exercise	Reps	Set	Weight	Notes

Notes

How many hours of sleep did I get?

Breakfast

Lunch

Dinner

Snacks

8oz 16oz 24oz 32oz 40oz 48oz 56oz 64oz

Macros

Carbs:

Energy Levels

Protein:

Fats:

Total Calories:

Resistance Workout Tracker

Exercise	Reps	Set	Weight	Notes

Cardio Workout Tracker

Exercise	Reps	Set	Weight	Notes

Notes

DAY 7

How many hours of sleep did I get?

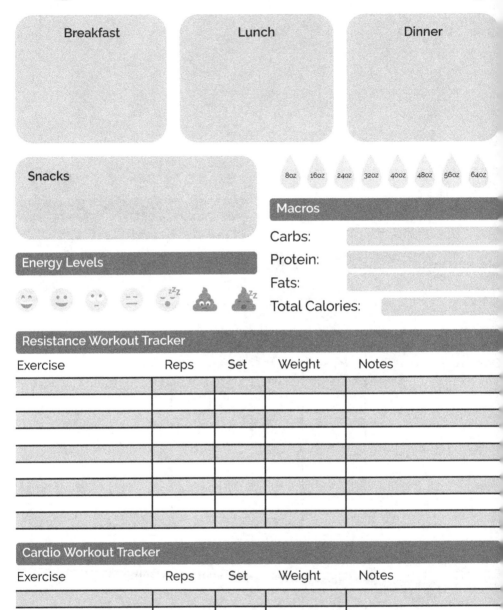

Breakfast	Lunch	Dinner

Snacks

8oz 16oz 24oz 32oz 40oz 48oz 56oz 64oz

Macros

Carbs:

Energy Levels

Protein:

Fats:

Total Calories:

Resistance Workout Tracker

Exercise	Reps	Set	Weight	Notes

Cardio Workout Tracker

Exercise	Reps	Set	Weight	Notes

Notes

How many hours of sleep did I get?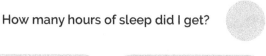

Breakfast

Lunch

Dinner

Snacks

8oz   16oz   24oz   32oz   40oz   48oz   56oz   64oz

Macros

Carbs:

Protein:

Fats:

Energy Levels

Total Calories:

Resistance Workout Tracker

Exercise	Reps	Set	Weight	Notes

Cardio Workout Tracker

Exercise	Reps	Set	Weight	Notes

Notes

DAY 9 How many hours of sleep did I get?

Breakfast	Lunch	Dinner

Snacks

8oz 16oz 24oz 32oz 40oz 48oz 56oz 64oz

Macros

Carbs:

Energy Levels

Protein:

Fats:

Total Calories:

Resistance Workout Tracker

Exercise	Reps	Set	Weight	Notes

Cardio Workout Tracker

Exercise	Reps	Set	Weight	Notes

Notes

How many hours of sleep did I get?

Breakfast

Lunch

Dinner

Snacks

8oz   16oz   24oz   32oz   40oz   48oz   56oz   64oz

Macros

Carbs:

Protein:

Fats:

Total Calories:

Energy Levels

    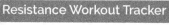

Resistance Workout Tracker

Exercise	Reps	Set	Weight	Notes

Cardio Workout Tracker

Exercise	Reps	Set	Weight	Notes

Notes

DAY 11   How many hours of sleep did I get?

Breakfast	Lunch	Dinner

Snacks

8oz 16oz 24oz 32oz 40oz 48oz 56oz 64oz

Macros

Carbs:

Protein:

Energy Levels

Fats:

Total Calories:

Resistance Workout Tracker

Exercise	Reps	Set	Weight	Notes

Cardio Workout Tracker

Exercise	Reps	Set	Weight	Notes

Notes

How many hours of sleep did I get?

Breakfast

Lunch

Dinner

Snacks

8oz 16oz 24oz 32oz 40oz 48oz 56oz 64oz

Macros

Carbs:

Energy Levels

Protein:

Fats:

Total Calories:

Resistance Workout Tracker

Exercise	Reps	Set	Weight	Notes

Cardio Workout Tracker

Exercise	Reps	Set	Weight	Notes

Notes

DAY 13   How many hours of sleep did I get?

Breakfast	Lunch	Dinner

Snacks

8oz 16oz 24oz 32oz 40oz 48oz 56oz 64oz

Macros

Energy Levels

Carbs:

Protein:

Fats:

Total Calories:

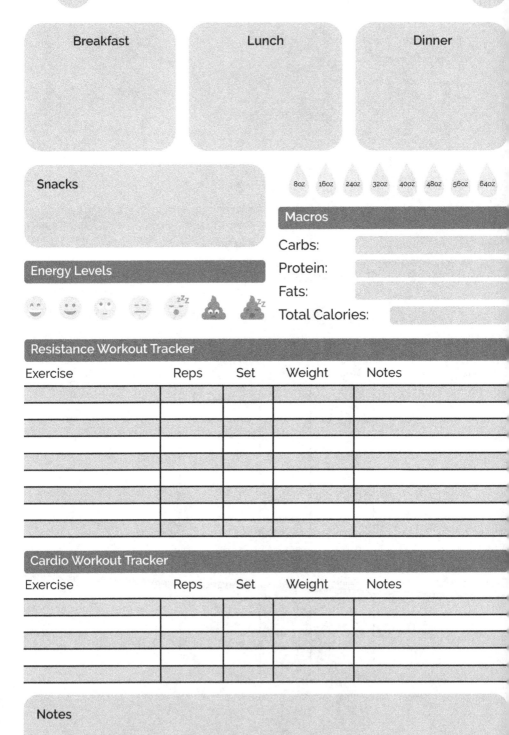

Resistance Workout Tracker

Exercise	Reps	Set	Weight	Notes

Cardio Workout Tracker

Exercise	Reps	Set	Weight	Notes

Notes

How many hours of sleep did I get?

Breakfast

Lunch

Dinner

Snacks

8oz 16oz 24oz 32oz 40oz 48oz 56oz 64oz

Macros

Carbs:

Protein:

Fats:

Total Calories:

Energy Levels

Resistance Workout Tracker

Exercise	Reps	Set	Weight	Notes

Cardio Workout Tracker

Exercise	Reps	Set	Weight	Notes

Notes

DAY 15

How many hours of sleep did I get?

Breakfast

Lunch

Dinner

Snacks

8oz 16oz 24oz 32oz 40oz 48oz 56oz 64oz

Macros

Carbs:

Energy Levels

Protein:

Fats:

Total Calories:

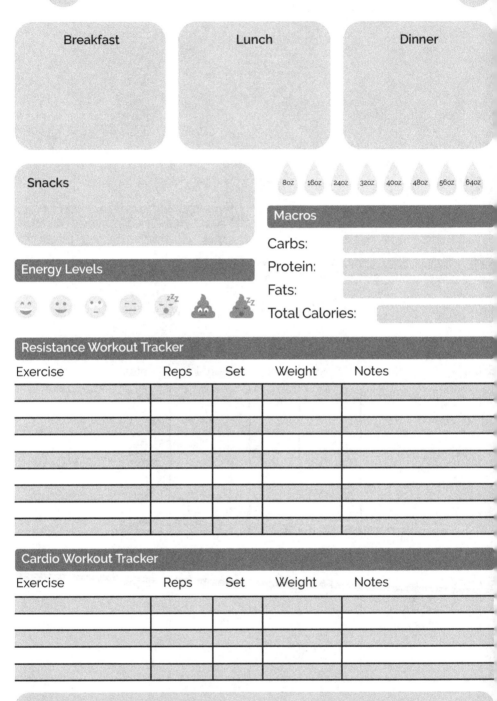

Resistance Workout Tracker

Exercise	Reps	Set	Weight	Notes

Cardio Workout Tracker

Exercise	Reps	Set	Weight	Notes

Notes

How many hours of sleep did I get?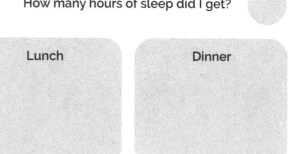

Breakfast

Lunch

Dinner

Snacks

8oz   16oz   24oz   32oz   40oz   48oz   56oz   64oz

Macros

Carbs:

Protein:

Fats:

Energy Levels

Total Calories:

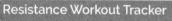

Resistance Workout Tracker

Exercise	Reps	Set	Weight	Notes

Cardio Workout Tracker

Exercise	Reps	Set	Weight	Notes

Notes

DAY 17   How many hours of sleep did I get?

Breakfast	Lunch	Dinner

Snacks

8oz 16oz 24oz 32oz 40oz 48oz 56oz 64oz

Macros

Carbs:

Energy Levels

Protein:

Fats:

Total Calories:

Resistance Workout Tracker

Exercise	Reps	Set	Weight	Notes

Cardio Workout Tracker

Exercise	Reps	Set	Weight	Notes

Notes

How many hours of sleep did I get?

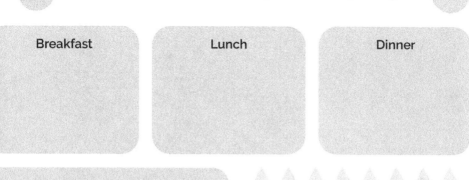

Breakfast	Lunch	Dinner

Snacks

8oz   16oz   24oz   32oz   40oz   48oz   56oz   64oz

Macros

Carbs:

Protein:

Fats:

Total Calories:

Energy Levels

Resistance Workout Tracker

Exercise	Reps	Set	Weight	Notes

Cardio Workout Tracker

Exercise	Reps	Set	Weight	Notes

Notes

DAY 19   How many hours of sleep did I get?

Breakfast	Lunch	Dinner

Snacks

8oz 16oz 24oz 32oz 40oz 48oz 56oz 64oz

Macros

Carbs:

Energy Levels

Protein:

Fats:

Total Calories:

Resistance Workout Tracker

Exercise	Reps	Set	Weight	Notes

Cardio Workout Tracker

Exercise	Reps	Set	Weight	Notes

Notes

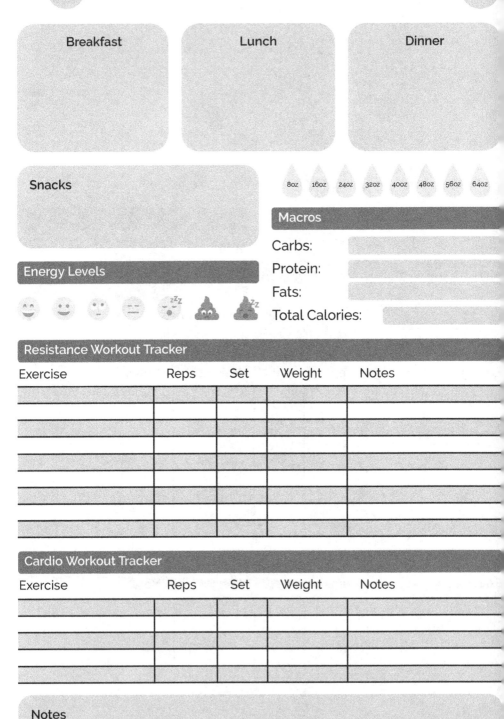

How many hours of sleep did I get?

Breakfast

Lunch

Dinner

Snacks

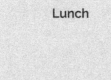

8oz 16oz 24oz 32oz 40oz 48oz 56oz 64oz

Macros

Energy Levels

Carbs:

Protein:

Fats:

Total Calories:

       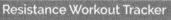

Resistance Workout Tracker

Exercise	Reps	Set	Weight	Notes

Cardio Workout Tracker

Exercise	Reps	Set	Weight	Notes

Notes

DAY 21   How many hours of sleep did I get?

Breakfast

Lunch

Dinner

Snacks

8oz   16oz   24oz   32oz   40oz   48oz   56oz   64oz

Macros

Carbs:

Protein:

Energy Levels

Fats:

Total Calories:

Resistance Workout Tracker

Exercise	Reps	Set	Weight	Notes

Cardio Workout Tracker

Exercise	Reps	Set	Weight	Notes

Notes

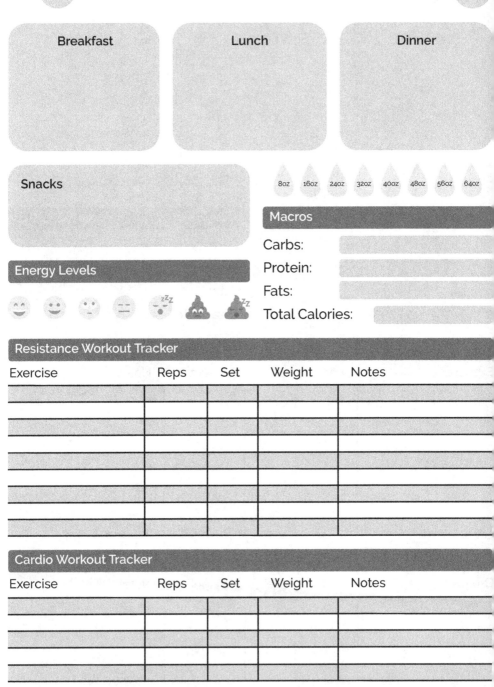

How many hours of sleep did I get?

Breakfast	Lunch	Dinner

Snacks

8oz 16oz 24oz 32oz 40oz 48oz 56oz 64oz

Macros

Carbs:

Protein:

Fats:

Total Calories:

Energy Levels

Resistance Workout Tracker

Exercise	Reps	Set	Weight	Notes

Cardio Workout Tracker

Exercise	Reps	Set	Weight	Notes

Notes

DAY 23

Breakfast	Lunch	Dinner

Snacks

8oz　16oz　24oz　32oz　40oz　48oz　56oz　64oz

Macros

Carbs:

Energy Levels

Protein:

Fats:

Total Calories:

Resistance Workout Tracker

Exercise	Reps	Set	Weight	Notes

Cardio Workout Tracker

Exercise	Reps	Set	Weight	Notes

Notes

How many hours of sleep did I get?

Breakfast

Lunch

Dinner

Snacks

8oz 16oz 24oz 32oz 40oz 48oz 56oz 64oz

Macros

Carbs:

Energy Levels

Protein:

Fats:

Total Calories:

Resistance Workout Tracker

Exercise	Reps	Set	Weight	Notes

Cardio Workout Tracker

Exercise	Reps	Set	Weight	Notes

Notes

DAY 25   How many hours of sleep did I get?

Breakfast	Lunch	Dinner

Snacks

8oz   16oz   24oz   32oz   40oz   48oz   56oz   64oz

Macros

Carbs:

Energy Levels

Protein:

Fats:

Total Calories:

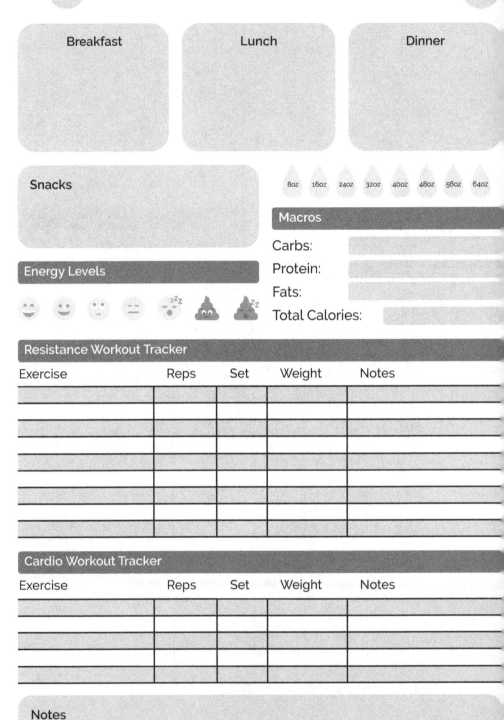

Resistance Workout Tracker

Exercise	Reps	Set	Weight	Notes

Cardio Workout Tracker

Exercise	Reps	Set	Weight	Notes

Notes

How many hours of sleep did I get?

Breakfast

Lunch

Dinner

Snacks

8oz   16oz   24oz   32oz   40oz   48oz   56oz   64oz

Macros

Carbs:

Protein:

Fats:

Total Calories:

Energy Levels

Resistance Workout Tracker

Exercise	Reps	Set	Weight	Notes

Cardio Workout Tracker

Exercise	Reps	Set	Weight	Notes

Notes

DAY 27   How many hours of sleep did I get?

Breakfast	Lunch	Dinner

Snacks

8oz 16oz 24oz 32oz 40oz 48oz 56oz 64oz

Macros

Carbs:

Protein:

Energy Levels

Fats:

Total Calories:

Resistance Workout Tracker

Exercise	Reps	Set	Weight	Notes

Cardio Workout Tracker

Exercise	Reps	Set	Weight	Notes

Notes

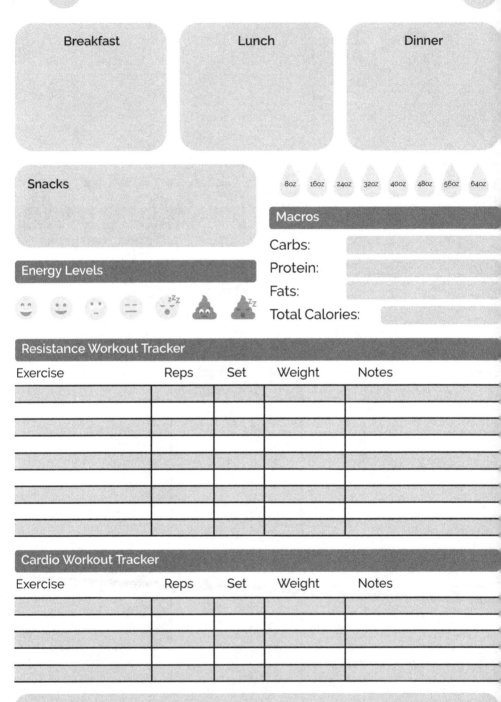

How many hours of sleep did I get?

Breakfast

Lunch

Dinner

Snacks

8oz 16oz 24oz 32oz 40oz 48oz 56oz 64oz

Macros

Carbs:

Protein:

Energy Levels

Fats:

Total Calories:

Resistance Workout Tracker

Exercise	Reps	Set	Weight	Notes

Cardio Workout Tracker

Exercise	Reps	Set	Weight	Notes

Notes

DAY 29   How many hours of sleep did I get?

Breakfast	Lunch	Dinner

Snacks

8oz   16oz   24oz   32oz   40oz   48oz   56oz   64oz

Macros

Carbs:

Protein:

Energy Levels

Fats:

Total Calories:

Resistance Workout Tracker

Exercise	Reps	Set	Weight	Notes

Cardio Workout Tracker

Exercise	Reps	Set	Weight	Notes

Notes

How many hours of sleep did I get?

Breakfast

Lunch

Dinner

Snacks

8oz   16oz   24oz   32oz   40oz   48oz   56oz   64oz

Macros

Carbs:

Energy Levels

Protein:

Fats:

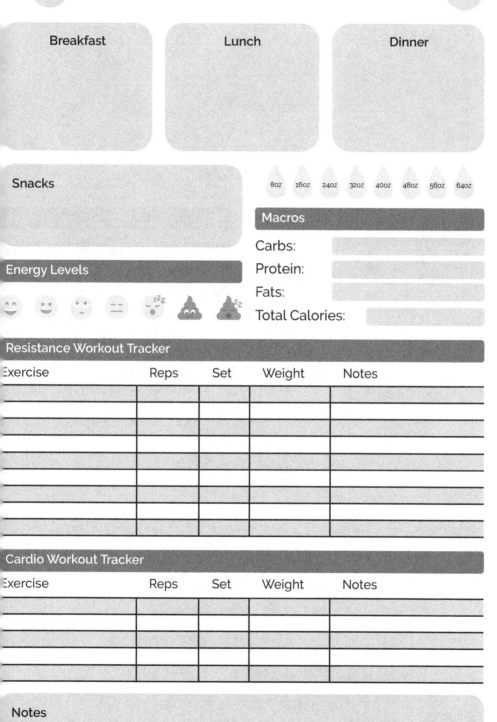

Total Calories:

Resistance Workout Tracker

Exercise	Reps	Set	Weight	Notes

Cardio Workout Tracker

Exercise	Reps	Set	Weight	Notes

Notes

DAY 31   How many hours of sleep did I get?

Breakfast

Lunch

Dinner

Snacks

8oz 16oz 24oz 32oz 40oz 48oz 56oz 64oz

Macros

Carbs:

Protein:

Energy Levels

Fats:

Total Calories:

Resistance Workout Tracker

Exercise	Reps	Set	Weight	Notes

Cardio Workout Tracker

Exercise	Reps	Set	Weight	Notes

Notes

How many hours of sleep did I get?

Breakfast

Lunch

Dinner

Snacks

8oz 16oz 24oz 32oz 40oz 48oz 56oz 64oz

Macros

Carbs:

Protein:

Fats:

Energy Levels

Total Calories:

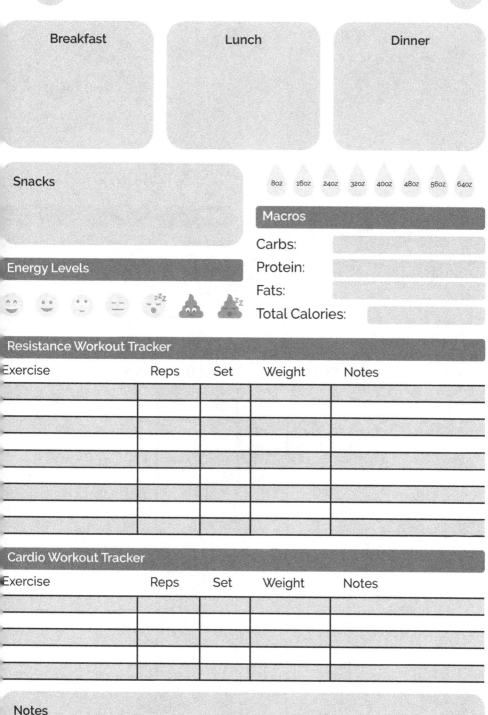

Resistance Workout Tracker

Exercise	Reps	Set	Weight	Notes

Cardio Workout Tracker

Exercise	Reps	Set	Weight	Notes

Notes

DAY 33

How many hours of sleep did I get?

Breakfast	Lunch	Dinner

Snacks

8oz   16oz   24oz   32oz   40oz   48oz   56oz   64oz

Macros

Carbs:

Energy Levels

Protein:

Fats:

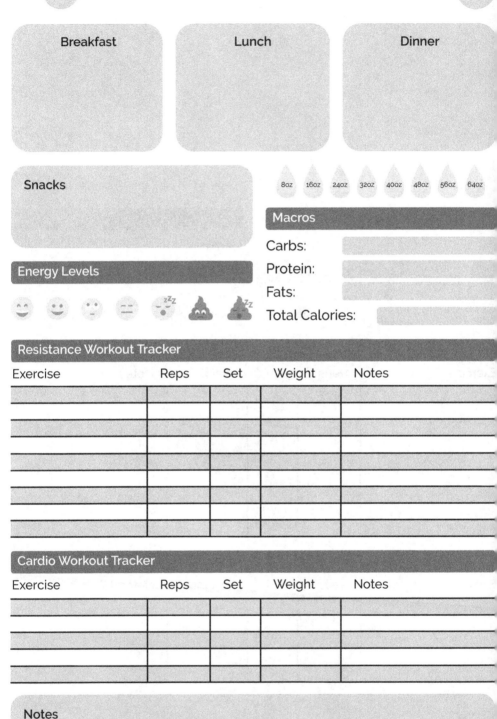

Total Calories:

Resistance Workout Tracker

Exercise	Reps	Set	Weight	Notes

Cardio Workout Tracker

Exercise	Reps	Set	Weight	Notes

Notes

How many hours of sleep did I get?

Breakfast

Lunch

Dinner

Snacks

8oz 16oz 24oz 32oz 40oz 48oz 56oz 64oz

Macros

Carbs:

Protein:

Fats:

Total Calories:

Energy Levels

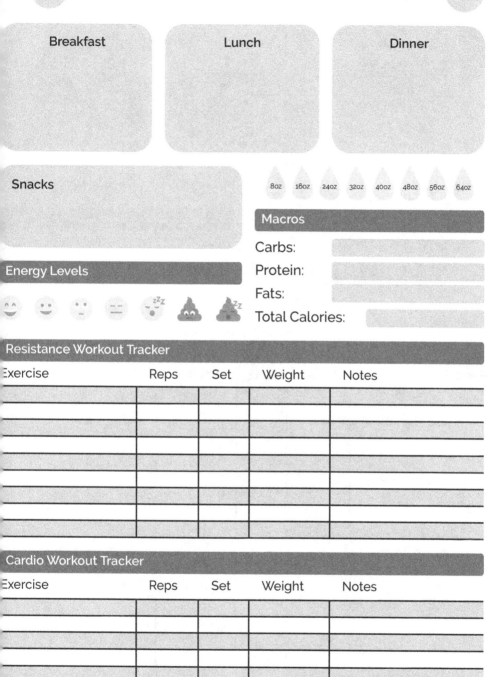

Resistance Workout Tracker

Exercise	Reps	Set	Weight	Notes

Cardio Workout Tracker

Exercise	Reps	Set	Weight	Notes

Notes

DAY 35   How many hours of sleep did I get?

Breakfast	Lunch	Dinner

Snacks

8oz   16oz   24oz   32oz   40oz   48oz   56oz   64oz

Macros

Carbs:

Protein:

Energy Levels

Fats:

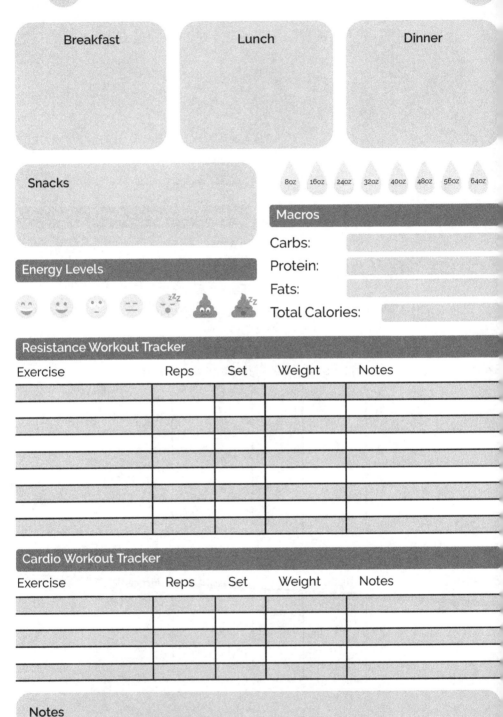

Total Calories:

Resistance Workout Tracker

Exercise	Reps	Set	Weight	Notes

Cardio Workout Tracker

Exercise	Reps	Set	Weight	Notes

Notes

How many hours of sleep did I get?

Breakfast

Lunch

Dinner

Snacks

8oz 16oz 24oz 32oz 40oz 48oz 56oz 64oz

Macros

Carbs:

Protein:

Energy Levels

Fats:

Total Calories:

Resistance Workout Tracker

Exercise	Reps	Set	Weight	Notes

Cardio Workout Tracker

Exercise	Reps	Set	Weight	Notes

Notes

DAY 37

How many hours of sleep did I get?

Breakfast	Lunch	Dinner

Snacks

8oz 16oz 24oz 32oz 40oz 48oz 56oz 64oz

Macros

Carbs:

Energy Levels

Protein:

Fats:

Total Calories:

Resistance Workout Tracker

Exercise	Reps	Set	Weight	Notes

Cardio Workout Tracker

Exercise	Reps	Set	Weight	Notes

Notes

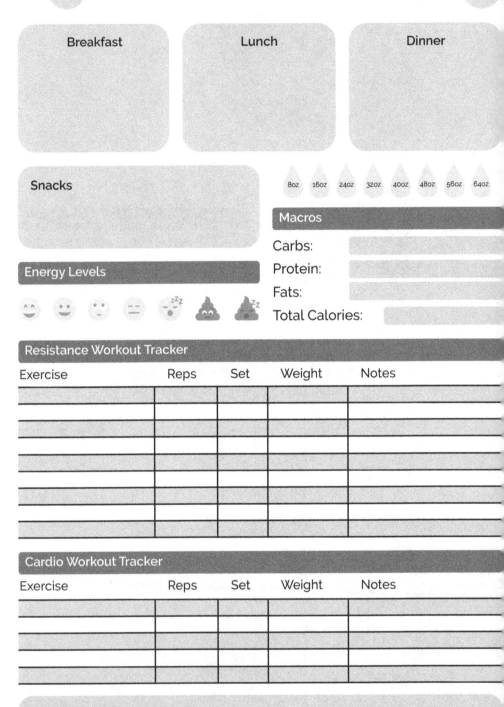

How many hours of sleep did I get?

Breakfast	Lunch	Dinner

Snacks

8oz 16oz 24oz 32oz 40oz 48oz 56oz 64oz

Macros

Carbs:

Energy Levels

Protein:

Fats:

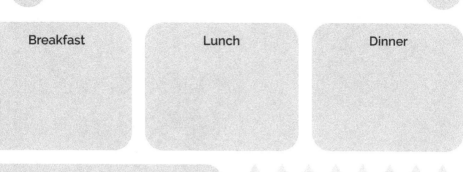

Total Calories:

Resistance Workout Tracker

Exercise	Reps	Set	Weight	Notes

Cardio Workout Tracker

Exercise	Reps	Set	Weight	Notes

Notes

DAY 39   How many hours of sleep did I get?

Breakfast

Lunch

Dinner

Snacks

8oz   16oz   24oz   32oz   40oz   48oz   56oz   64oz

Macros

Carbs:

Protein:

Energy Levels

Fats:

Total Calories:

Resistance Workout Tracker

Exercise	Reps	Set	Weight	Notes

Cardio Workout Tracker

Exercise	Reps	Set	Weight	Notes

Notes

How many hours of sleep did I get?

Breakfast	Lunch	Dinner

Snacks

8oz   16oz   24oz   32oz   40oz   48oz   56oz   64oz

Macros

Carbs:

Energy Levels

Protein:

Fats:

Total Calories:

Resistance Workout Tracker

Exercise	Reps	Set	Weight	Notes

Cardio Workout Tracker

Exercise	Reps	Set	Weight	Notes

Notes

DAY 41

How many hours of sleep did I get?

Breakfast	Lunch	Dinner

Snacks

8oz   16oz   24oz   32oz   40oz   48oz   56oz   64oz

Macros

Carbs:

Energy Levels

Protein:

Fats:

Total Calories:

Resistance Workout Tracker

Exercise	Reps	Set	Weight	Notes

Cardio Workout Tracker

Exercise	Reps	Set	Weight	Notes

Notes

How many hours of sleep did I get?

Breakfast	Lunch	Dinner

Snacks

8oz 16oz 24oz 32oz 40oz 48oz 56oz 64oz

Macros

Carbs:

Protein:

Fats:

Total Calories:

Energy Levels

Resistance Workout Tracker

Exercise	Reps	Set	Weight	Notes

Cardio Workout Tracker

Exercise	Reps	Set	Weight	Notes

Notes

DAY 43

How many hours of sleep did I get?

Breakfast

Lunch

Dinner

Snacks

8oz 16oz 24oz 32oz 40oz 48oz 56oz 64oz

Carbs:

Protein:

Energy Levels

Fats:

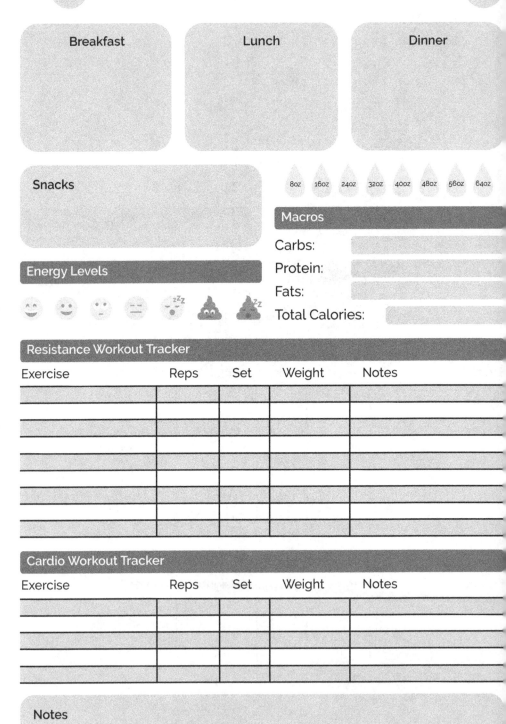

Total Calories:

Resistance Workout Tracker

Exercise	Reps	Set	Weight	Notes

Cardio Workout Tracker

Exercise	Reps	Set	Weight	Notes

Notes

How many hours of sleep did I get?

Breakfast

Lunch

Dinner

Snacks

8oz 16oz 24oz 32oz 40oz 48oz 56oz 64oz

Macros

Carbs:

Protein:

Fats:

Total Calories:

Energy Levels

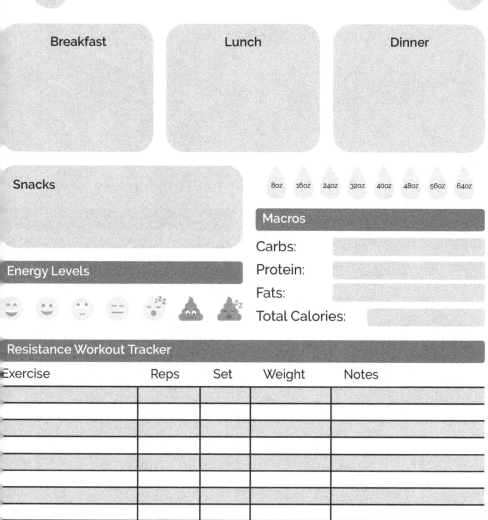

Resistance Workout Tracker

Exercise	Reps	Set	Weight	Notes

Cardio Workout Tracker

Exercise	Reps	Set	Weight	Notes

Notes

DAY 45

How many hours of sleep did I get?

Breakfast	Lunch	Dinner

Snacks

8oz   16oz   24oz   32oz   40oz   48oz   56oz   64oz

Macros

Carbs:

Protein:

Energy Levels

Fats:

Total Calories:

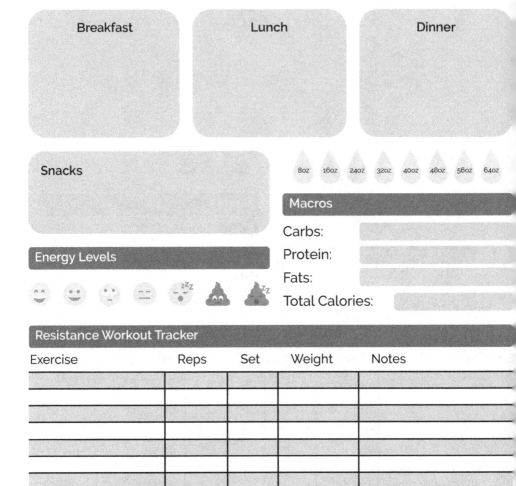

Resistance Workout Tracker

Exercise	Reps	Set	Weight	Notes

Cardio Workout Tracker

Exercise	Reps	Set	Weight	Notes

Notes

Let's Keep Going!

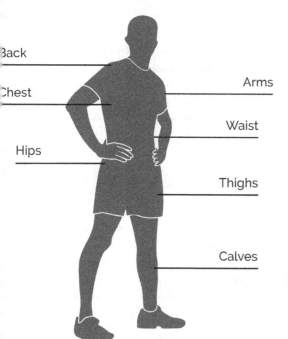

Back

Chest

Arms

Waist

Hips

Thighs

Calves

Weight: _____

Heart Rate: _____

Blood Pressure: _____

Back

Chest

Arms

Waist

Hips

Thighs

Calves

Weight: _____

Heart Rate: _____

Blood Pressure: _____

DAY 46   How many hours of sleep did I get?

Breakfast	Lunch	Dinner

Snacks

8oz 16oz 24oz 32oz 40oz 48oz 56oz 64oz

Macros

Carbs:

Protein:

Energy Levels

Fats:

Total Calories:

Resistance Workout Tracker

Exercise	Reps	Set	Weight	Notes

Cardio Workout Tracker

Exercise	Reps	Set	Weight	Notes

Notes

How many hours of sleep did I get?

Breakfast	Lunch	Dinner

Snacks

8oz 16oz 24oz 32oz 40oz 48oz 56oz 64oz

Macros

Carbs:

Protein:

Energy Levels

Fats:

Total Calories:

Resistance Workout Tracker

Exercise	Reps	Set	Weight	Notes

Cardio Workout Tracker

Exercise	Reps	Set	Weight	Notes

Notes

DAY 48   How many hours of sleep did I get?

Breakfast	Lunch	Dinner

Snacks

8oz   16oz   24oz   32oz   40oz   48oz   56oz   64oz

Macros

Energy Levels

Carbs:

Protein:

Fats:

Total Calories:

Resistance Workout Tracker

Exercise	Reps	Set	Weight	Notes

Cardio Workout Tracker

Exercise	Reps	Set	Weight	Notes

Notes

How many hours of sleep did I get?

Breakfast

Lunch

Dinner

Snacks

8oz   16oz   24oz   32oz   40oz   48oz   56oz   64oz

Macros

Carbs:

Energy Levels

Protein:

Fats:

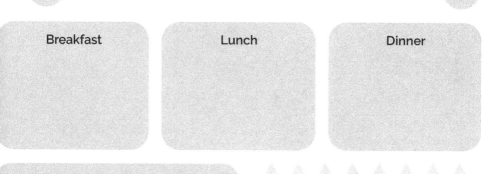

Total Calories:

Resistance Workout Tracker

Exercise	Reps	Set	Weight	Notes

Cardio Workout Tracker

Exercise	Reps	Set	Weight	Notes

Notes

How many hours of sleep did I get?

Breakfast	Lunch	Dinner

Snacks

8oz 16oz 24oz 32oz 40oz 48oz 56oz 64oz

Macros

Carbs:

Energy Levels

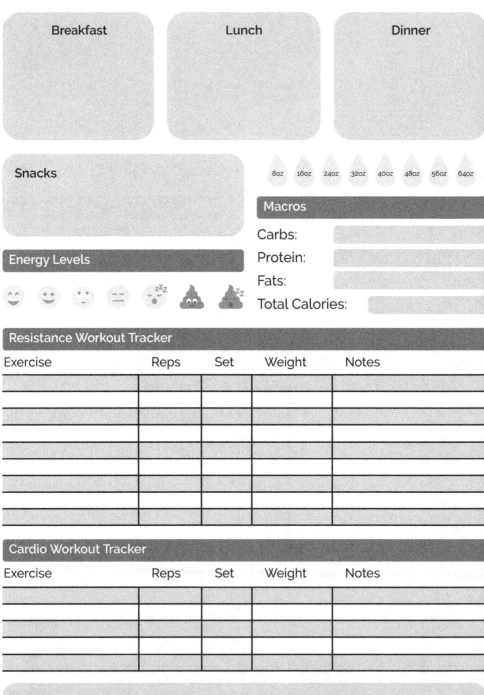

Protein:

Fats:

Total Calories:

Resistance Workout Tracker

Exercise	Reps	Set	Weight	Notes

Cardio Workout Tracker

Exercise	Reps	Set	Weight	Notes

Notes

How many hours of sleep did I get?

Breakfast

Lunch

Dinner

Snacks

8oz 16oz 24oz 32oz 40oz 48oz 56oz 64oz

Macros

Carbs:

Energy Levels

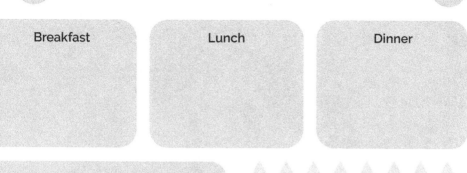

Protein:

Fats:

Total Calories:

Resistance Workout Tracker

Exercise	Reps	Set	Weight	Notes

Cardio Workout Tracker

Exercise	Reps	Set	Weight	Notes

Notes

How many hours of sleep did I get?

Breakfast

Lunch

Dinner

Snacks

8oz   16oz   24oz   32oz   40oz   48oz   56oz   64oz

Macros

Carbs:

Protein:

Fats:

Energy Levels

Total Calories:

Resistance Workout Tracker

Exercise	Reps	Set	Weight	Notes

Cardio Workout Tracker

Exercise	Reps	Set	Weight	Notes

Notes

How many hours of sleep did I get?

Breakfast	Lunch	Dinner

Snacks

8oz 16oz 24oz 32oz 40oz 48oz 56oz 64oz

Macros

Carbs:

Energy Levels

Protein:

Fats:

Total Calories:

Resistance Workout Tracker

Exercise	Reps	Set	Weight	Notes

Cardio Workout Tracker

Exercise	Reps	Set	Weight	Notes

Notes

DAY 54   How many hours of sleep did I get?

Breakfast	Lunch	Dinner

Snacks

8oz 16oz 24oz 32oz 40oz 48oz 56oz 64oz

Macros

Carbs:

Energy Levels

Protein:

Fats:

Total Calories:

Resistance Workout Tracker

Exercise	Reps	Set	Weight	Notes

Cardio Workout Tracker

Exercise	Reps	Set	Weight	Notes

Notes

How many hours of sleep did I get?

Breakfast

Lunch

Dinner

Snacks

8oz 16oz 24oz 32oz 40oz 48oz 56oz 64oz

Macros

Carbs:

Protein:

Fats:

Total Calories:

Energy Levels

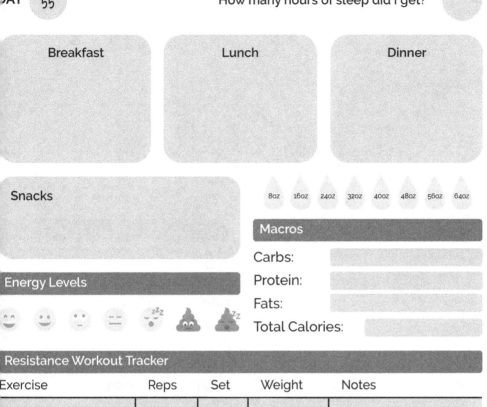

Resistance Workout Tracker

Exercise	Reps	Set	Weight	Notes

Cardio Workout Tracker

Exercise	Reps	Set	Weight	Notes

Notes

How many hours of sleep did I get?

Breakfast

Lunch

Dinner

Snacks

8oz 16oz 24oz 32oz 40oz 48oz 56oz 64oz

Macros

Carbs:

Energy Levels

Protein:

Fats:

Total Calories:

Resistance Workout Tracker

Exercise	Reps	Set	Weight	Notes

Cardio Workout Tracker

Exercise	Reps	Set	Weight	Notes

Notes

How many hours of sleep did I get?

Breakfast

Lunch

Dinner

Snacks

8oz 16oz 24oz 32oz 40oz 48oz 56oz 64oz

Macros

Carbs:

Protein:

Fats:

Total Calories:

Energy Levels

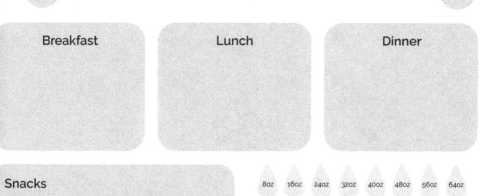

Resistance Workout Tracker

Exercise	Reps	Set	Weight	Notes

Cardio Workout Tracker

Exercise	Reps	Set	Weight	Notes

Notes

DAY 58   How many hours of sleep did I get?

Breakfast	Lunch	Dinner

Snacks

8oz   16oz   24oz   32oz   40oz   48oz   56oz   64oz

Macros

Carbs:

Energy Levels

Protein:

Fats:

Total Calories:

Resistance Workout Tracker

Exercise	Reps	Set	Weight	Notes

Cardio Workout Tracker

Exercise	Reps	Set	Weight	Notes

Notes

How many hours of sleep did I get?

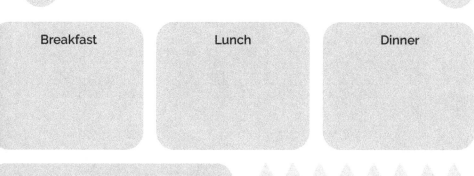

Breakfast

Lunch

Dinner

Snacks

8oz 16oz 24oz 32oz 40oz 48oz 56oz 64oz

Macros

Carbs:

Protein:

Energy Levels

Fats:

Total Calories:

Resistance Workout Tracker

Exercise	Reps	Set	Weight	Notes

Cardio Workout Tracker

Exercise	Reps	Set	Weight	Notes

Notes

DAY 60   How many hours of sleep did I get?

Breakfast	Lunch	Dinner

Snacks

8oz   16oz   24oz   32oz   40oz   48oz   56oz   64oz

Macros

Carbs:

Protein:

Energy Levels

Fats:

Total Calories:

Resistance Workout Tracker

Exercise	Reps	Set	Weight	Notes

Cardio Workout Tracker

Exercise	Reps	Set	Weight	Notes

Notes

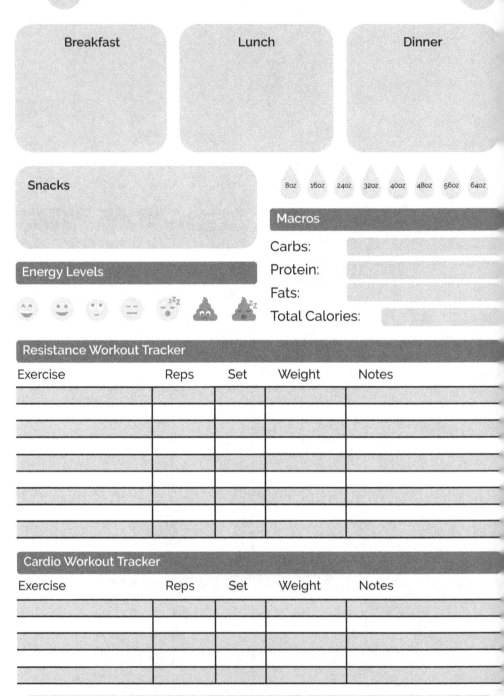

How many hours of sleep did I get?

Breakfast

Lunch

Dinner

Snacks

8oz 16oz 24oz 32oz 40oz 48oz 56oz 64oz

Macros

Carbs:

Protein:

Energy Levels

Fats:

Total Calories:

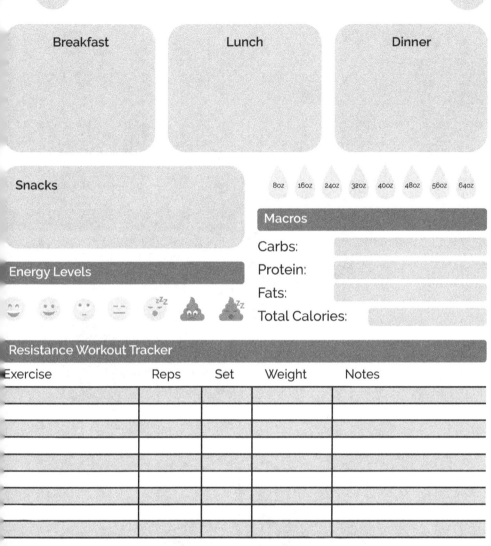

Resistance Workout Tracker

Exercise	Reps	Set	Weight	Notes

Cardio Workout Tracker

Exercise	Reps	Set	Weight	Notes

Notes

How many hours of sleep did I get?

Breakfast	Lunch	Dinner

Snacks

8oz　16oz　24oz　32oz　40oz　48oz　56oz　64oz

Macros

Carbs:

Energy Levels

Protein:

Fats:

Total Calories:

Resistance Workout Tracker

Exercise	Reps	Set	Weight	Notes

Cardio Workout Tracker

Exercise	Reps	Set	Weight	Notes

Notes

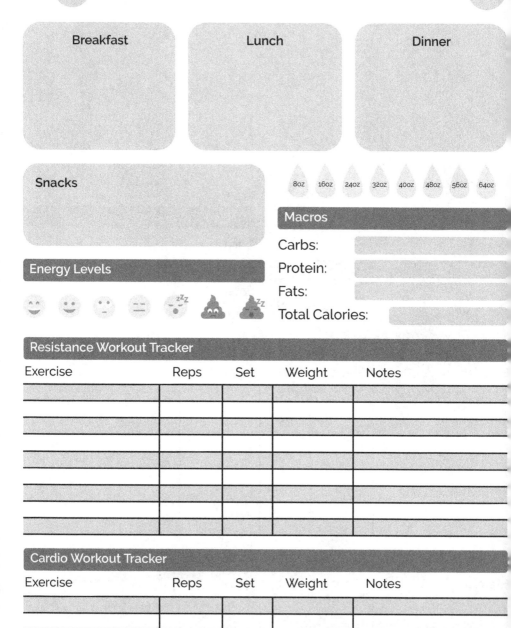

How many hours of sleep did I get?

Breakfast

Lunch

Dinner

Snacks

8oz 16oz 24oz 32oz 40oz 48oz 56oz 64oz

Macros

Carbs:

Protein:

Fats:

Total Calories:

Energy Levels

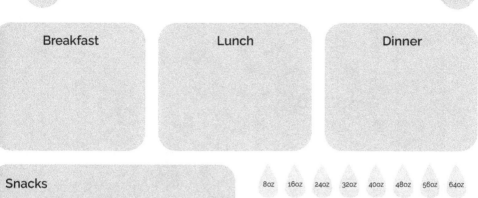

Resistance Workout Tracker

Exercise	Reps	Set	Weight	Notes

Cardio Workout Tracker

Exercise	Reps	Set	Weight	Notes

Notes

DAY 64   How many hours of sleep did I get?

Breakfast	Lunch	Dinner

Snacks

8oz 16oz 24oz 32oz 40oz 48oz 56oz 64oz

Macros

Carbs:

Energy Levels

Protein:

Fats:

Total Calories:

Resistance Workout Tracker

Exercise	Reps	Set	Weight	Notes

Cardio Workout Tracker

Exercise	Reps	Set	Weight	Notes

Notes

How many hours of sleep did I get?

Breakfast

Lunch

Dinner

Snacks

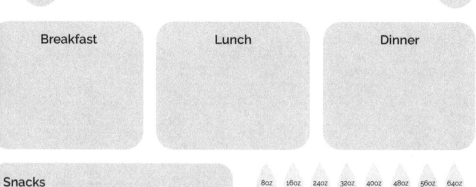

8oz　16oz　24oz　32oz　40oz　48oz　56oz　64oz

Macros

Carbs:

Protein:

Fats:

Total Calories:

Energy Levels

Resistance Workout Tracker

Exercise	Reps	Set	Weight	Notes

Cardio Workout Tracker

Exercise	Reps	Set	Weight	Notes

Notes

How many hours of sleep did I get?

Breakfast

Lunch

Dinner

Snacks

8oz 16oz 24oz 32oz 40oz 48oz 56oz 64oz

Macros

Carbs:

Protein:

Fats:

Total Calories:

Energy Levels

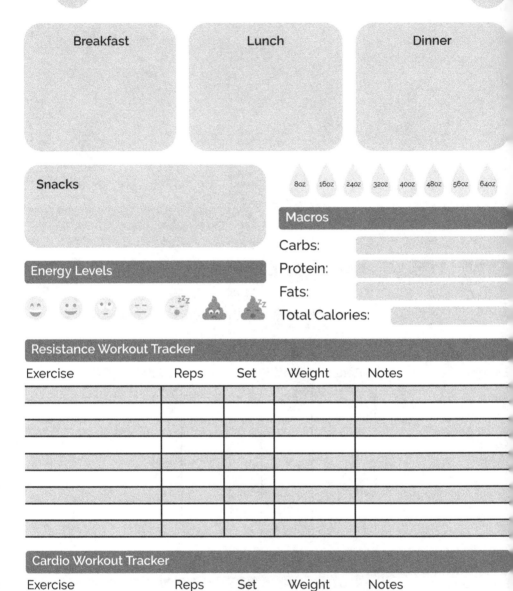

Resistance Workout Tracker

Exercise	Reps	Set	Weight	Notes

Cardio Workout Tracker

Exercise	Reps	Set	Weight	Notes

Notes

How many hours of sleep did I get?

Breakfast

Lunch

Dinner

Snacks

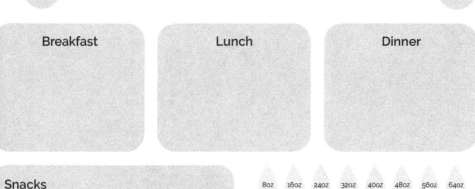

8oz 16oz 24oz 32oz 40oz 48oz 56oz 64oz

Macros

Carbs:

Protein:

Fats:

Total Calories:

Energy Levels

Resistance Workout Tracker

Exercise	Reps	Set	Weight	Notes

Cardio Workout Tracker

Exercise	Reps	Set	Weight	Notes

Notes

DAY 68

How many hours of sleep did I get?

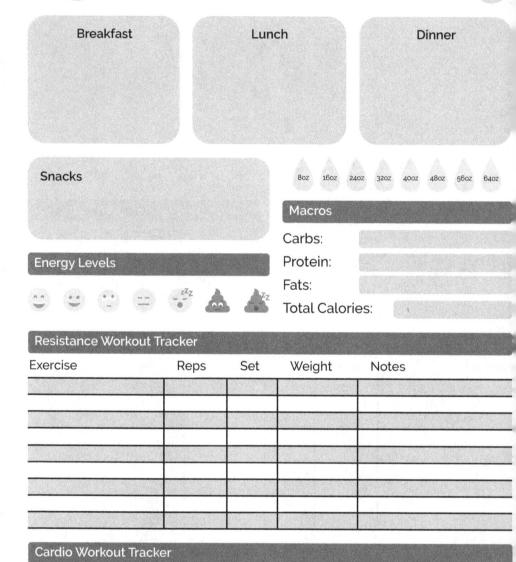

Breakfast

Lunch

Dinner

Snacks

8oz 16oz 24oz 32oz 40oz 48oz 56oz 64oz

Macros

Carbs:

Protein:

Fats:

Total Calories:

Energy Levels

Resistance Workout Tracker

Exercise	Reps	Set	Weight	Notes

Cardio Workout Tracker

Exercise	Reps	Set	Weight	Notes

Notes

How many hours of sleep did I get?

Breakfast	Lunch	Dinner

Snacks

8oz 16oz 24oz 32oz 40oz 48oz 56oz 64oz

Macros

Carbs:

Protein:

Fats:

Total Calories:

Energy Levels

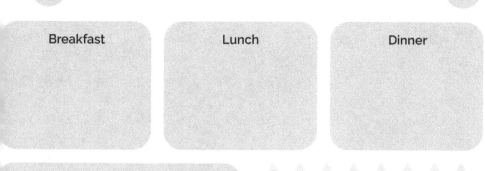

Resistance Workout Tracker

Exercise	Reps	Set	Weight	Notes

Cardio Workout Tracker

Exercise	Reps	Set	Weight	Notes

Notes

DAY 70 How many hours of sleep did I get?

Breakfast	Lunch	Dinner

Snacks

8oz 16oz 24oz 32oz 40oz 48oz 56oz 64oz

Macros

Carbs:

Protein:

Energy Levels

Fats:

Total Calories:

Resistance Workout Tracker

Exercise	Reps	Set	Weight	Notes

Cardio Workout Tracker

Exercise	Reps	Set	Weight	Notes

Notes

How many hours of sleep did I get?

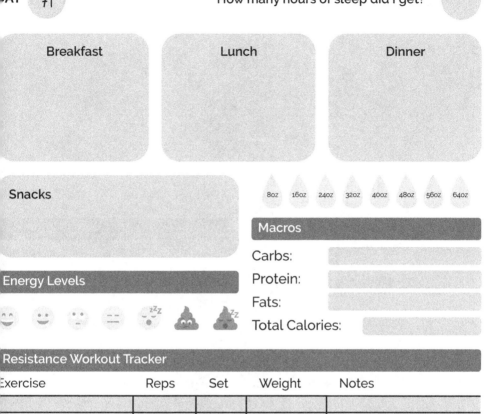

Breakfast

Lunch

Dinner

Snacks

8oz 16oz 24oz 32oz 40oz 48oz 56oz 64oz

Macros

Carbs:

Protein:

Fats:

Total Calories:

Energy Levels

Resistance Workout Tracker

Exercise	Reps	Set	Weight	Notes

Cardio Workout Tracker

Exercise	Reps	Set	Weight	Notes

Notes

DAY 72   How many hours of sleep did I get?

Breakfast	Lunch	Dinner

Snacks

8oz 16oz 24oz 32oz 40oz 48oz 56oz 64oz

Macros

Carbs:

Protein:

Fats:

Energy Levels

Total Calories:

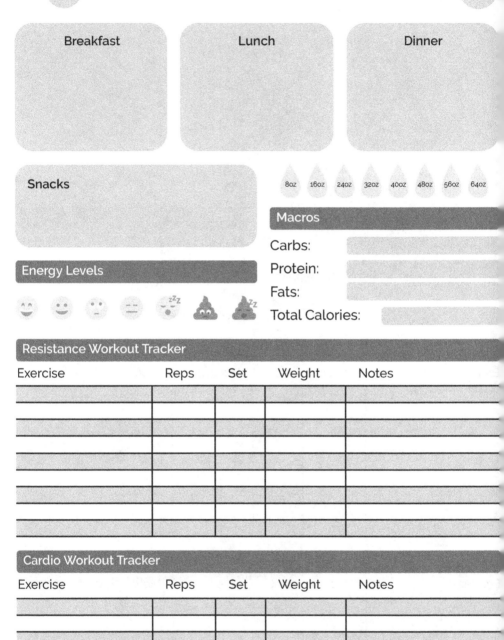

Resistance Workout Tracker

Exercise	Reps	Set	Weight	Notes

Cardio Workout Tracker

Exercise	Reps	Set	Weight	Notes

Notes

How many hours of sleep did I get?

Breakfast

Lunch

Dinner

Snacks

8oz 16oz 24oz 32oz 40oz 48oz 56oz 64oz

Macros

Carbs:

Protein:

Energy Levels

Fats:

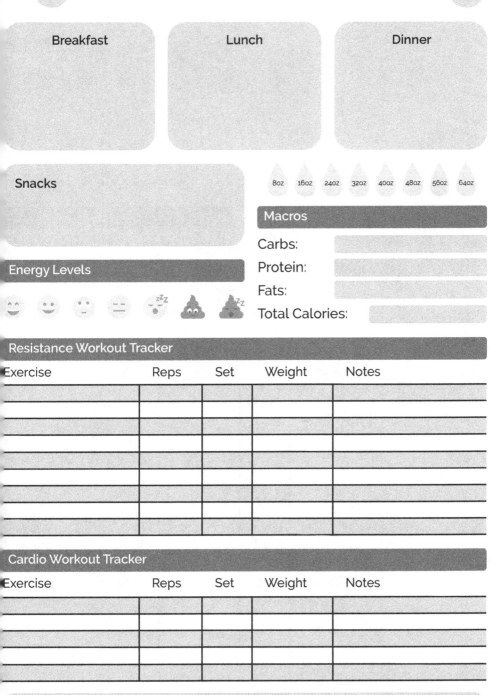

Total Calories:

Resistance Workout Tracker

Exercise	Reps	Set	Weight	Notes

Cardio Workout Tracker

Exercise	Reps	Set	Weight	Notes

Notes

How many hours of sleep did I get?

Breakfast

Lunch

Dinner

Snacks

8oz   16oz   24oz   32oz   40oz   48oz   56oz   64oz

Macros

Carbs:

Protein:

Fats:

Total Calories:

Energy Levels

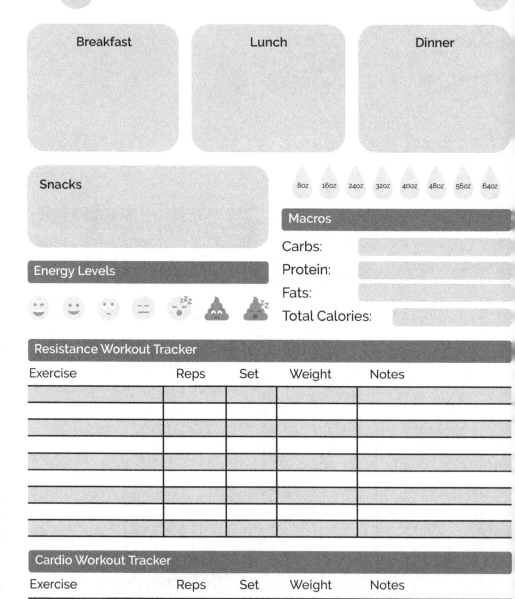

Resistance Workout Tracker

Exercise	Reps	Set	Weight	Notes

Cardio Workout Tracker

Exercise	Reps	Set	Weight	Notes

Notes

How many hours of sleep did I get?

Breakfast

Lunch

Dinner

Snacks

8oz 16oz 24oz 32oz 40oz 48oz 56oz 64oz

Macros

Carbs:

Protein:

Fats:

Total Calories:

Energy Levels

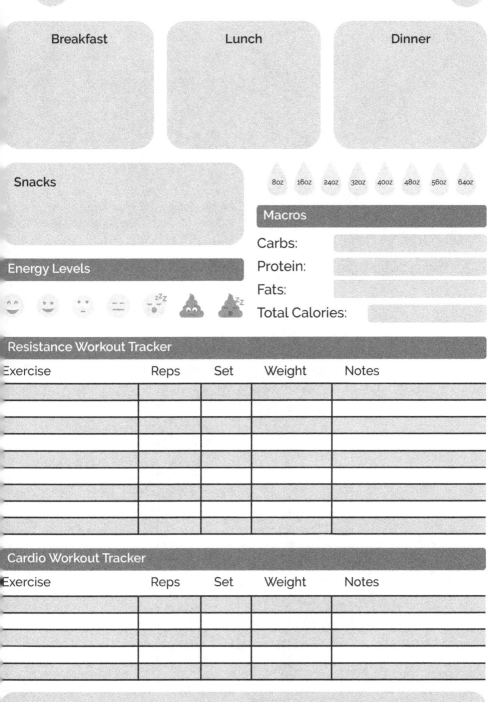

Resistance Workout Tracker

Exercise	Reps	Set	Weight	Notes

Cardio Workout Tracker

Exercise	Reps	Set	Weight	Notes

Notes

How many hours of sleep did I get?

Breakfast	Lunch	Dinner

Snacks

8oz 16oz 24oz 32oz 40oz 48oz 56oz 64oz

Macros

Carbs:

Protein:

Energy Levels

Fats:

Total Calories:

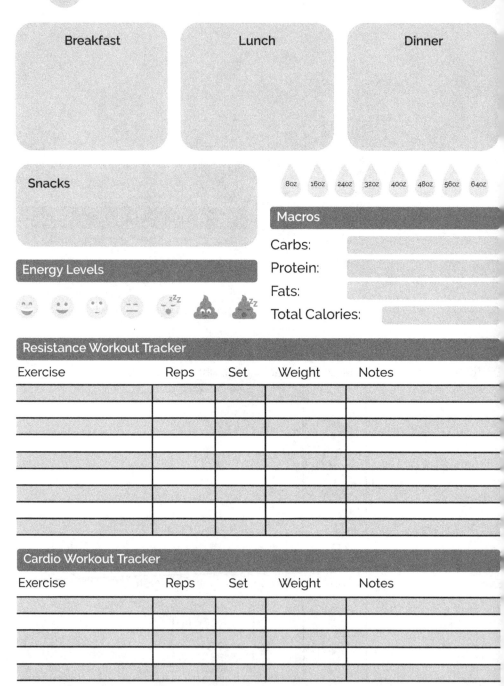

Resistance Workout Tracker

Exercise	Reps	Set	Weight	Notes

Cardio Workout Tracker

Exercise	Reps	Set	Weight	Notes

Notes

How many hours of sleep did I get?

Breakfast	Lunch	Dinner

Snacks

8oz 16oz 24oz 32oz 40oz 48oz 56oz 64oz

Macros

Carbs:

Protein:

Fats:

Total Calories:

Energy Levels

Resistance Workout Tracker

Exercise	Reps	Set	Weight	Notes

Cardio Workout Tracker

Exercise	Reps	Set	Weight	Notes

Notes

DAY 78   How many hours of sleep did I get?

Breakfast	Lunch	Dinner

Snacks

8oz 16oz 24oz 32oz 40oz 48oz 56oz 64oz

Macros

Carbs:

Energy Levels

Protein:

Fats:

Total Calories:

Resistance Workout Tracker

Exercise	Reps	Set	Weight	Notes

Cardio Workout Tracker

Exercise	Reps	Set	Weight	Notes

Notes

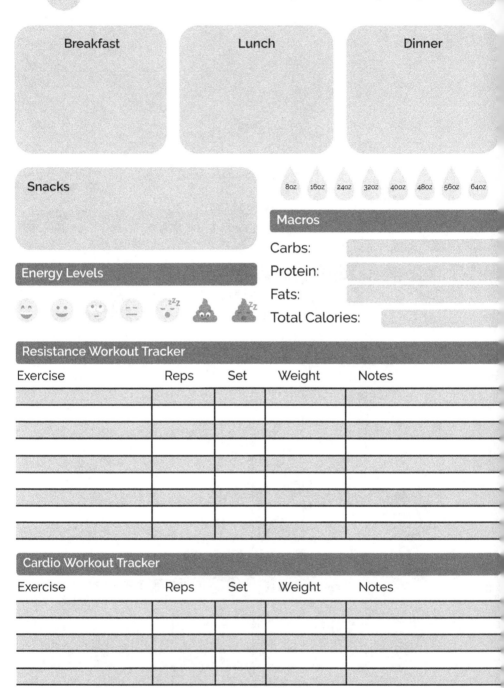

How many hours of sleep did I get?

Breakfast

Lunch

Dinner

Snacks

8oz 16oz 24oz 32oz 40oz 48oz 56oz 64oz

Macros

Carbs:

Protein:

Fats:

Total Calories:

Energy Levels

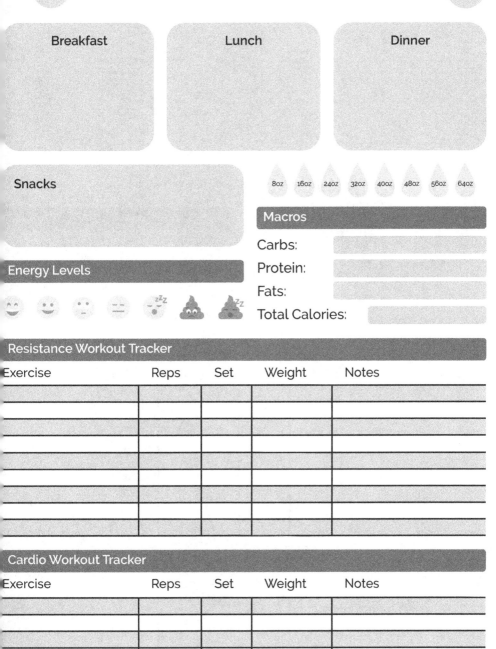

Resistance Workout Tracker

Exercise	Reps	Set	Weight	Notes

Cardio Workout Tracker

Exercise	Reps	Set	Weight	Notes

Notes

DAY 80

How many hours of sleep did I get?

Breakfast

Lunch

Dinner

Snacks

8oz 16oz 24oz 32oz 40oz 48oz 56oz 64oz

Macros

Carbs:

Energy Levels

Protein:

Fats:

Total Calories:

Resistance Workout Tracker

Exercise	Reps	Set	Weight	Notes

Cardio Workout Tracker

Exercise	Reps	Set	Weight	Notes

Notes

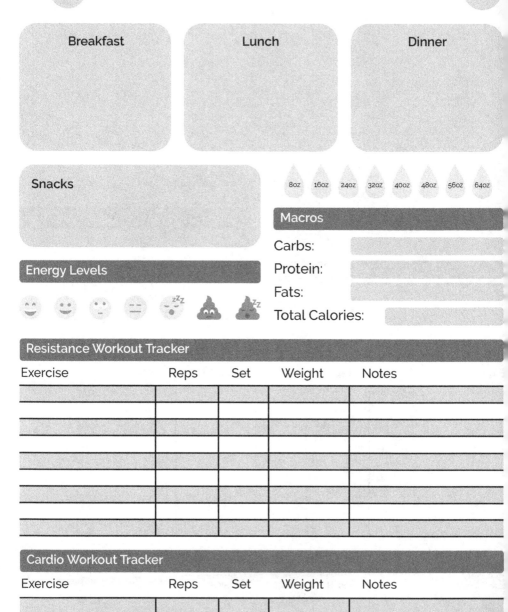

How many hours of sleep did I get?

Breakfast	Lunch	Dinner

Snacks

8oz 16oz 24oz 32oz 40oz 48oz 56oz 64oz

Macros

Carbs:

Protein:

Fats:

Total Calories:

Energy Levels

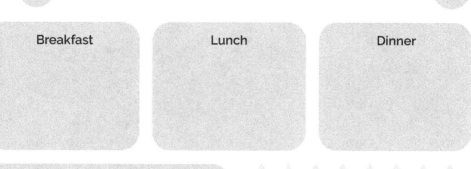

Resistance Workout Tracker

Exercise	Reps	Set	Weight	Notes

Cardio Workout Tracker

Exercise	Reps	Set	Weight	Notes

Notes

DAY 82

How many hours of sleep did I get?

Breakfast	Lunch	Dinner

Snacks

8oz 16oz 24oz 32oz 40oz 48oz 56oz 64oz

Macros

Carbs:

Energy Levels

Protein:

Fats:

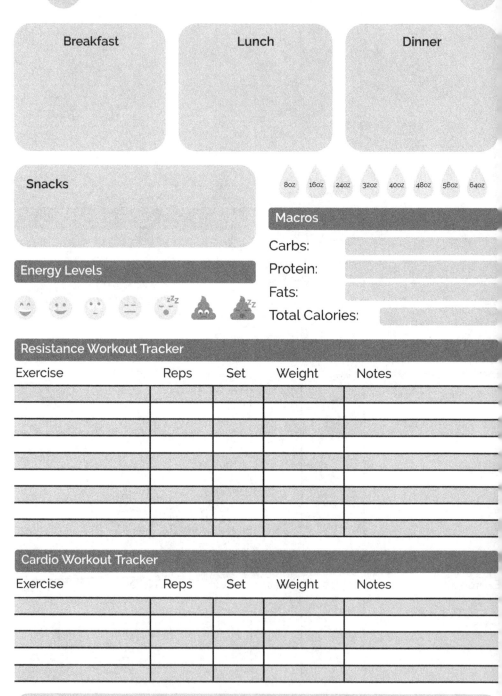

Total Calories:

Resistance Workout Tracker

Exercise	Reps	Set	Weight	Notes

Cardio Workout Tracker

Exercise	Reps	Set	Weight	Notes

Notes

How many hours of sleep did I get?

Breakfast

Lunch

Dinner

Snacks

8oz 16oz 24oz 32oz 40oz 48oz 56oz 64oz

Macros

Carbs:

Energy Levels

Protein:

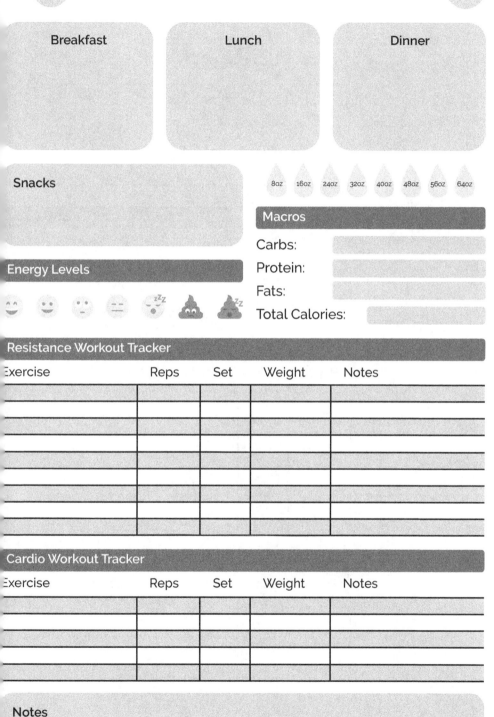

Fats:

Total Calories:

Resistance Workout Tracker

Exercise	Reps	Set	Weight	Notes

Cardio Workout Tracker

Exercise	Reps	Set	Weight	Notes

Notes

How many hours of sleep did I get?

Breakfast	Lunch	Dinner

Snacks

8oz 16oz 24oz 32oz 40oz 48oz 56oz 64oz

Macros

Carbs:

Energy Levels

Protein:

Fats:

Total Calories:

Resistance Workout Tracker

Exercise	Reps	Set	Weight	Notes

Cardio Workout Tracker

Exercise	Reps	Set	Weight	Notes

Notes

How many hours of sleep did I get?

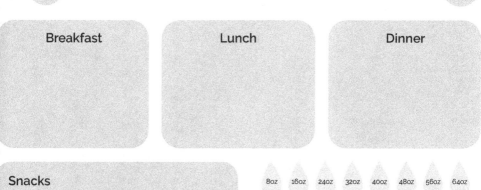

Breakfast

Lunch

Dinner

Snacks

8oz 16oz 24oz 32oz 40oz 48oz 56oz 64oz

Macros

Carbs:

Protein:

Energy Levels

Fats:

Total Calories:

Resistance Workout Tracker

Exercise	Reps	Set	Weight	Notes

Cardio Workout Tracker

Exercise	Reps	Set	Weight	Notes

Notes

DAY 86

How many hours of sleep did I get?

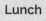

Breakfast

Lunch

Dinner

Snacks

8oz 16oz 24oz 32oz 40oz 48oz 56oz 64oz

Macros

Carbs:

Protein:

Fats:

Total Calories:

Energy Levels

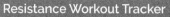

Resistance Workout Tracker

Exercise	Reps	Set	Weight	Notes

Cardio Workout Tracker

Exercise	Reps	Set	Weight	Notes

Notes

How many hours of sleep did I get?

Breakfast

Lunch

Dinner

Snacks

8oz 16oz 24oz 32oz 40oz 48oz 56oz 64oz

Macros

Carbs:

Protein:

Fats:

Energy Levels

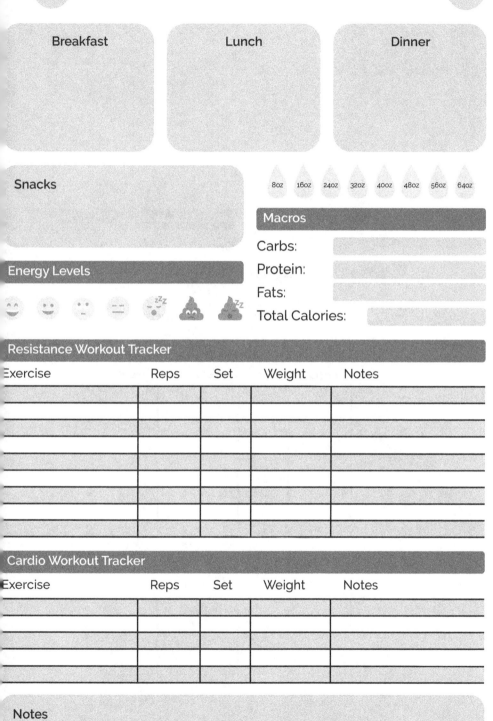

Total Calories:

Resistance Workout Tracker

Exercise	Reps	Set	Weight	Notes

Cardio Workout Tracker

Exercise	Reps	Set	Weight	Notes

Notes

DAY 88   How many hours of sleep did I get?

Breakfast	Lunch	Dinner

Snacks

8oz 16oz 24oz 32oz 40oz 48oz 56oz 64oz

Macros

Carbs:

Protein:

Fats:

Energy Levels

zZz   Zz

Total Calories:

Resistance Workout Tracker

Exercise	Reps	Set	Weight	Notes

Cardio Workout Tracker

Exercise	Reps	Set	Weight	Notes

Notes

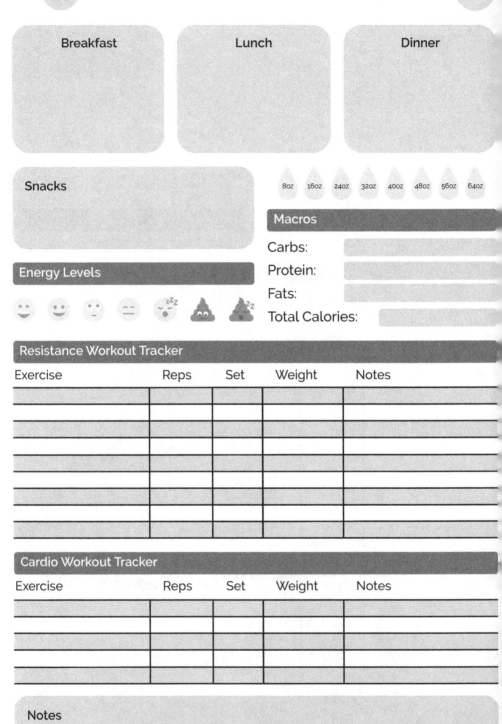

How many hours of sleep did I get?

Breakfast

Lunch

Dinner

Snacks

8oz 16oz 24oz 32oz 40oz 48oz 56oz 64oz

Macros

Carbs:

Protein:

Fats:

Total Calories:

Energy Levels

Resistance Workout Tracker

Exercise	Reps	Set	Weight	Notes

Cardio Workout Tracker

Exercise	Reps	Set	Weight	Notes

Notes

How many hours of sleep did I get?

Breakfast	Lunch	Dinner

Snacks

8oz 16oz 24oz 32oz 40oz 48oz 56oz 64oz

Macros

Carbs:

Energy Levels

Protein:

Fats:

Total Calories:

Resistance Workout Tracker

Exercise	Reps	Set	Weight	Notes

Cardio Workout Tracker

Exercise	Reps	Set	Weight	Notes

Notes

Look How Far You've Come!

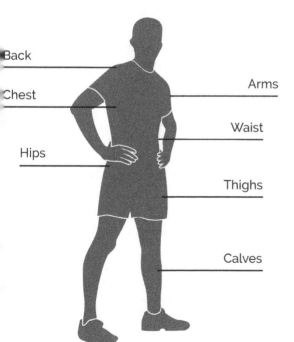

Back

Chest

Hips

Arms

Waist

Thighs

Calves

Back

Arms

Chest

Waist

Hips

Thighs

Calves

Weight: _____

Heart Rate: _____

Blood Pressure: _____

Weight: _____

Heart Rate: _____

Blood Pressure: _____

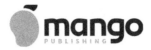

Mango Publishing, established in 2014, publishes an eclectic list of books by diverse authors—both new and established voices—on topics ranging from business, personal growth, women's empowerment, LGBTQ studies, health, and spirituality to history, popular culture, time management, decluttering, lifestyle, mental wellness, aging, and sustainable living. We were recently named 2019's #1 fastest growing independent publisher by *Publishers Weekly.* Our success is driven by our main goal, which is to publish high quality books that will entertain readers as well as make a positive difference in their lives.

Our readers are our most important resource; we value your input, suggestions, and ideas. We'd love to hear from you—after all, we are publishing books for you.

Please stay in touch with us and follow us at:

Facebook: Mango Publishing

Twitter: @MangoPublishing

Instagram: @MangoPublishing

LinkedIn: Mango Publishing

Pinterest: Mango Publishing

Sign up for our newsletter at www.mango.bz and receive a free book.

Join us on Mango's journey to reinvent publishing, one book at a time.

CPSIA information can be obtained
at www.ICGtesting.com
Printed in the USA
BVHW041446011119
562696BV00001B/1/P